Contents

INTRODUCTION

Diabetes Mellitus ("diabetes" for short) is a serious disease that occurs when your body has difficulty properly regulating the amount of dissolved sugar (glucose) in your blood stream. It is unrelated to a similarly named disorder "Diabetes Insipidus" which involves kidney-related fluid retention problems.

In order to understand diabetes, it is necessary to first understand the role glucose plays with regard to the body, and what can happen when regulation of glucose fails and blood sugar levels become dangerously low or high.

The tissues and cells that make up the human body are living things, and require food to stay alive. The food cells eat is a type of sugar called glucose. Fixed in place as they are, the body's cells are completely dependent on the blood stream in which they are bathed to bring glucose to them. Without access to adequate glucose, the body's cells have nothing to fuel themselves with and soon die.

Human beings eat food, not glucose. Human foods get converted into glucose as a part of the normal digestion process. Once converted, glucose enters the blood stream, causing the level of dissolved glucose inside the blood to rise. The blood stream then carries the dissolved glucose to the various tissues and cells of the body.

Though glucose may be available in the blood, nearby cells are not able to access that glucose without the aid of a chemical hormone called insulin. Insulin acts as a key to open the cells, allowing them to receive and utilize available glucose. Cells absorb glucose from the blood in the presence of insulin, and blood sugar levels drop as sugar leaves the blood and enters the cells. Insulin can be thought of as a bridge for glucose between the blood stream and cells. It is important to understand when levels of insulin increase, levels of sugar in the blood decrease (because the sugar goes into the cells to be used for energy).

The body is designed to regulate and buffer the amount of glucose dissolved in the blood to maintain a steady supply to meet cell needs. The pancreas, one of your body's many organs, produces, stores and releases insulin into the blood stream to bring glucose levels back down.

The concentration of glucose available in the blood stream at any given moment is dependent on the amount and type of foods that people eat. Refined carbohydrates, candy and sweets are easy to break down into glucose. Correspondingly, blood glucose levels rise rapidly after such foods have been eaten. In contrast, blood sugars rises gradually and slowly after eating more complex, unrefined carbohydrates (oatmeal, apples, baked potatoes, etc.) which require more digestive steps take place before glucose can be yielded. Faced with rapidly rising blood glucose concentrations, the body must react quickly by releasing large amounts of insulin all at once or risk a dangerous condition called Hyperglycemia (high blood sugar) which will be described below. The influx of insulin enables cells to utilize glucose, and glucose concentrations drop. While glucose levels can rise and fall rapidly, insulin levels change much more slowly. When a large amount of simple sugar is eaten the bloodstream quickly becomes flooded with glucose. Insulin is released by the pancreas in response to the increased sugar. The glucose rapidly enters the cells but the high levels of insulin remain in the bloodstream for a period of time. This can result in an overabundance of insulin in the blood, which can trigger feelings of hunger and even Hypoglycemia (low blood sugar), another serious condition. When blood glucose concentrations rise more gradually, there is less need for dramatic compensation. Insulin can be released in a more controlled and safer manner which requires the body experience less strain. This more gradual process will leave you feeling "full" or content for a longer period of time. For these reasons, it is best for overall health to limit the amount and frequency of sweets and refined sugars in your diet. Instead eat more complex sugars such as raw fruit, whole wheat bread and pasta, and beans. The difference between simple and complex sugars (carbohydrates) is exemplified by the difference between white (simple) and whole wheat (more complex) bread.

Insulin is the critical key to the cell's ability to use glucose. Problems with insulin production or with how insulin is recognized by the cells can easily cause the body's carefully balanced glucose metabolism system to get out of control. When either of these problems occur, Diabetes develops, blood sugar levels surge and crash and the body risks becoming damaged.

Key facts

The number of people with diabetes rose from 108 million in 1980 to 422 million in 2014.

The global prevalence of diabetes* among adults over 18 years of age rose from 4.7% in 1980 to 8.5% in 2014.

Between 2000 and 2016, there was a 5% increase in premature mortality from diabetes.

Diabetes prevalence has been rising more rapidly in low- and middle-income countries than in high-income countries.

Diabetes is a major cause of blindness, kidney failure, heart attacks, stroke and lower limb amputation.

In 2016, an estimated 1.6 million deaths were directly caused by diabetes. Another 2.2 million deaths were attributable to high blood glucose in 2012.

Almost half of all deaths attributable to high blood glucose occur before the age of 70 years. WHO estimates that diabetes was the seventh leading cause of death in 2016.

A healthy diet, regular physical activity, maintaining a normal body weight and avoiding tobacco use are ways to prevent or delay the onset of type 2 diabetes.

Diabetes can be treated and its consequences avoided or delayed with diet, physical activity, medication and regular screening and treatment for complications.

Overview

Diabetes is a chronic disease that occurs either when the pancreas does not produce enough insulin or when the body cannot effectively use the insulin it produces. Insulin is a hormone that regulates blood sugar. Hyperglycaemia, or raised blood sugar, is a common effect of uncontrolled diabetes and over time leads to serious damage to many of the body's systems, especially the nerves and blood vessels.

In 2014, 8.5% of adults aged 18 years and older had diabetes. In 2016, diabetes was the direct cause of 1.6 million deaths and in 2012 high blood glucose was the cause of another 2.2 million deaths.

Between 2000 and 2016, there was a 5% increase in premature mortality from diabetes. In high-income countries the premature mortality rate due to diabetes decreased from 2000 to 2010 but then increased in 2010-2016. In lower-middle-income countries, the premature mortality rate due to diabetes increased across both periods.

By contrast, the probability of dying from any one of the four main noncommunicable diseases (cardiovascular diseases, cancer, chronic respiratory diseases or diabetes) between the ages of 30 and 70 decreased by 18% globally between 2000 and 2016.

CHAPTER ONE

What is Diabetes?

Diabetes is a disease that occurs when your blood glucose, also called blood sugar, is too high. Blood glucose is your main source of energy and comes from the food you eat. Insulin, a hormone made by the pancreas, helps glucose from food get into your cells to be used for energy. Sometimes your body doesn't make enough—or any—insulin or doesn't use insulin well. Glucose then stays in your blood and doesn't reach your cells.

Over time, having too much glucose in your blood can cause health problems. Although diabetes has no cure, you can take steps to manage your diabetes and stay healthy.

Sometimes people call diabetes "a touch of sugar" or "borderline diabetes." These terms suggest that someone doesn't really have diabetes or has a less serious case, but every case of diabetes is serious.

What are the different types of diabetes?

The most common types of diabetes are type 1, type 2, and gestational diabetes.

Type 1 diabetes

If you have type 1 diabetes, your body does not make insulin. Your immune system attacks and destroys the cells in your pancreas that make insulin. Type 1 diabetes is usually diagnosed in children and young adults, although it can appear at any age. People with type 1 diabetes need to take insulin every day to stay alive.

Type 2 diabetes

If you have type 2 diabetes, your body does not make or use insulin well. You can develop type 2 diabetes at any age, even during childhood. However, this type of diabetes occurs most often in middle-aged and older people. Type 2 is the most common type of diabetes.

Gestational diabetes

Gestational diabetes develops in some women when they are pregnant. Most of the time, this type of diabetes goes away after the baby is born. However, if you've had gestational diabetes, you have a greater chance of developing type 2 diabetes later in life. Sometimes diabetes diagnosed during pregnancy is actually type 2 diabetes.

Other types of diabetes

Less common types include monogenic diabetes, which is an inherited form of diabetes, and cystic fibrosis-related diabetes External link.

Causes of diabetes

Different causes are associated with each type of diabetes.

Type 1 diabetes

Doctors don't know exactly what causes type 1 diabetes. For some reason, the immune system mistakenly attacks and destroys insulin-producing beta cells in the pancreas.

Genes may play a role in some people. It's also possible that a virus sets off the immune system attack.

Type 2 diabetes

Type 2 diabetes stems from a combination of genetics and lifestyle factors. Being overweight or obese increases your risk too. Carrying extra weight, especially in your belly, makes your cells more resistant to the effects of insulin on your blood sugar.

This condition runs in families. Family members share genes that make them more likely to get type 2 diabetes and to be overweight.

Gestational diabetes

Gestational diabetes is the result of hormonal changes during pregnancy. The placenta produces hormones that make a pregnant woman's cells less sensitive to the effects of insulin. This can cause high blood sugar during pregnancy.

Women who are overweight when they get pregnant or who gain too much weight during their pregnancy are more likely to get gestational diabetes.

How does Type 2 diabetes affect your heart?

After we eat, we begin to digest foods and break carbohydrates down into glucose. In people who don't have diabetes, insulin is released by their pancreas when they eat. It acts as a signal for cells around their body to absorb the glucose and use it as fuel for energy.

If you have Type 2 diabetes, your body doesn't make enough insulin or can't use the insulin it makes, and the cells don't absorb enough glucose. This causes high levels of glucose in your bloodstream.

High levels of glucose in your blood can damage the walls of your arteries, and make them more likely to develop fatty deposits (atheroma).

If atheroma builds up in your coronary arteries (the arteries that supply oxygen-rich blood to your heart), this is coronary heart disease and can lead to a heart attack. If this happens in the arteries that carry blood to your brain it can lead to a stroke.

What are the signs and symptoms of Type 2 diabetes?

It's not always easy to tell if you have diabetes. Many people with Type 2 diabetes have no symptoms and don't know they have it, or symptoms can develop slowly or start out of the blue - it varies from person to person.

You may have diabetes if you are:

often very thirsty

peeing more than usual, particularly at night

often very tired

losing weight unexpectedly

having blurred vision

having genital itching or regular episodes of thrush

noticing that your cuts or wounds heal slowly.

Don't ignore symptoms. Your doctor can diagnose you, help you manage your condition and stop things getting worse.

Is there a difference between the signs of type 1 and type 2 diabetes?

Type 1 diabetes normally onsets in childhood. Type 2 normally onsets in adulthood, over the age of 30. Type 1 is not associated with excess body weight; type 2 is often associated with excess weight. Type 1 is often associated with higher levels of ketone during diagnosis; type 2 is often associated with high blood pressure and cholesterol level during diagnosis.

Diabetes risk factors

Certain factors increase your risk for diabetes.

Type 1 diabetes

You're more likely to get type 1 diabetes if you're a child or teenager, you have a parent or sibling with the condition, or you carry certain genes that are linked to the disease.

Type 2 diabetes

Your risk for type 2 diabetes increases if you:

are overweight

are age 45 or older

have a parent or sibling with the condition

aren't physically active

have had gestational diabetes

have prediabetes

have high blood pressure, high cholesterol, or high triglycerides have African American, Hispanic or Latino American, Alaska Native, Pacific Islander, American Indian, or Asian American ancestry

Gestational diabetes

Gestational diabetes

Your risk for gestational diabetes increases if you:

are overweight

are over age 25

had gestational diabetes during a past pregnancy

have given birth to a baby weighing more than 9 pounds

have a family history of type 2 diabetes

have polycystic ovary syndrome (PCOS)

Diabetes complications

Over a long period of time, high glucose levels in your blood can seriously damage your heart, your eyes, your feet and your kidneys. These are known as the complications of diabetes.

But with the right treatment and care, people can live a healthy life. And there's much less risk that someone will experience these complications.

Find out more about the different types of complications, and what you can do to reduce your risk of developing them.

How is Type 2 diabetes diagnosed?

If you have any of the symptoms listed above, contact your GP. They may arrange a blood test to check your blood glucose level and they may also test your urine.

Finger-prick blood glucose levels can be taken, or there is a blood test called an HbA1c (Haemoglobin A1c) that is used to test what your average blood glucose has been over a few months. It can be more helpful for doctors as it gives them a long term view of what your blood glucose level is, whereas a finger-prick blood glucose can only test what your blood sugar is at that very moment.

How common is diabetes?

As of 2015, 30.3 million people in the United States, or 9.4 percent of the population, had diabetes. More than 1 in 4 of them didn't know they had the disease. Diabetes affects 1 in 4 people over the age of 65. About 90-95 percent of cases in adults are type 2 diabetes.

Who is more likely to develop type 2 diabetes?

You are more likely to develop type 2 diabetes if you are age 45 or older, have a family history of diabetes, or are overweight. Physical inactivity, race, and certain health problems such as high blood pressure also affect your chance of developing type 2 diabetes. You are also more likely to develop type 2 diabetes if you have prediabetes or had gestational diabetes when you were pregnant. Learn more about risk factors for type 2 diabetes.

What health problems can people with diabetes develop?

Over time, high blood glucose leads to problems such as

heart disease

stroke

kidney disease

eye problems

dental disease

nerve damage

foot problems

You can take steps to lower your chances of developing these diabetes-related health problems.

How can a GP test for type 2 diabetes?

"The most useful way to screen for type 2 diabetes would be to ask your GP for an HbA1c blood test," says Dr Woodhouse. Glucose in the blood sticks to HbA1C – a type of haemoglobin found in red blood cells.

She adds: "A level of 48mmol/L would indicate type 2 diabetes but anything in the range 42-47mmol/L is a marker for pre-diabetes. This is far more accurate in understanding a person's long term (last three months) blood sugar control. In addition, it can pick up pre-diabetes."

How can I manage my Type 2 diabetes?

If you have diabetes, it's very important to make sure that you control your blood glucose levels, blood pressure and cholesterol levels to help reduce your risk of heart and circulatory diseases like coronary heart disease, heart attack and stroke. You can do this by managing your weight and sticking to a healthy lifestyle.

Your doctor will regularly check your HbA1c (haemoglobin A1c) levels and you will review them together to see how stable your glucose level has been over a period of time. These levels will help your doctor work out whether your lifestyle changes and medication are working, or if they need to make a change to your treatment plan. If your treatment plan has changed you may have an HbA1c test after 3 months, and once you are stable on a treatment plan your HbA1c levels need to be checked every 6 months.

Diabetes prevention

Type 1 diabetes isn't preventable because it's caused by a problem with the immune system. Some causes of type 2 diabetes, such as your genes or age, aren't under your control either.

Yet many other diabetes risk factors are controllable. Most diabetes prevention strategies involve making simple adjustments to your diet and fitness routine.

If you've been diagnosed with prediabetes, here are a few things you can do to delay or prevent type 2 diabetes:

Get at least 150 minutes per week of aerobic exercise, such as walking or cycling.

Cut saturated and trans fats, along with refined carbohydrates, out of your diet.

Eat more fruits, vegetables, and whole grains.

Eat smaller portions.

Try to lose 7 percentTrusted Source of your body weight if you're overweight or obese.

These aren't the only ways to prevent diabetes. Discover more strategies that may help you avoid this chronic disease.

Diabetes in pregnancy

Women who've never had diabetes can suddenly develop gestational diabetes in pregnancy. Hormones produced by the placenta can make your body more resistant to the effects of insulin.

Some women who had diabetes before they conceived carry it with them into pregnancy. This is called pre-gestational diabetes.

Gestational diabetes should go away after you deliver, but it does significantly increase your risk for getting diabetes later.

About half of women with gestational diabetes will develop type 2 diabetes within 5 to 10 years of delivery, according to the International Diabetes Federation (IDF).

Having diabetes during your pregnancy can also lead to complications for your newborn, such as jaundice or breathing problems.

If you're diagnosed with pre-gestational or gestational diabetes, you'll need special monitoring to prevent complications. Find out more about the effect of diabetes on pregnancy.

Diabetes in children

Children can get both type 1 and type 2 diabetes. Controlling blood sugar is especially important in young people, because the disease can damage important organs such as the heart and kidneys.

Type 1 diabetes

The autoimmune form of diabetes often starts in childhood. One of the main symptoms is increased urination. Kids with type 1 diabetes may start wetting the bed after they've been toilet trained.

Extreme thirst, fatigue, and hunger are also signs of the condition. It's important that children with type 1 diabetes get treated right away. The disease can cause high blood sugar and dehydration, which can be medical emergencies.

Type 2 diabetes

Type 1 diabetes used to be called "juvenile diabetes" because type 2 was so rare in children. Now that more children are overweight or obese, type 2 diabetes is becoming more common in this age group.

About 40 percent of children with type 2 diabetes don't have symptoms, according to the Mayo Clinic. The disease is often diagnosed during a physical exam.

Untreated type 2 diabetes can cause lifelong complications, including heart disease, kidney disease, and blindness. Healthy eating and exercise can help your child manage their blood sugar and prevent these problems.

Type 2 diabetes is more prevalent than ever in young people. Learn how to spot the signs so you can report them to your child's doctor.

Medications and treatments for Type 2 diabetes

You can manage diabetes very successfully with lifestyle changes and medicines. The first line of treatment if you're overweight is to try and lose some weight, become more physically active, and have a healthy diet -

including cutting down on sugary and fatty foods and drinks.

If this doesn't help to control your glucose levels, your doctor may prescribe medication such as Metformin and Sitagliptin. Type 2 diabetes can progress over the years and so treatment may change over time. Many people with Type 2 diabetes eventually need to have insulin injections to control their diabetes.

Type 2 diabetes puts you at higher risk of having a heart attack or stroke, so your doctor may prescribe a cholesterol-lowering medicine such as statins to help protect your heart. Your doctor may also recommend that you take a fibrate medicine to help control your triglyceride levels.

If you have diabetes, you should have a review each year with your GP or diabetes nurse to make sure that you're not developing any of the complications of diabetes, including coronary heart disease.

What are the three most common symptoms of undiagnosed diabetes?

Frequent need to pee, especially at night; tiredness and thirst

Can diabetes go away on its own?

Diabetes can't be permanently cured and won't go away of its own accord. But it can be controlled with the right lifestyle and drugs, so you can lead a normal life.

What is diabetic ketoacidosis?

Diabetic ketoacidosis occurs in people with diabetes when the body begins to run out of insulin and starts to break down fat for energy instead of glucose.

While diabetic ketoacidosis usually occurs in people with Type 1 diabetes, it can occasionally happen to people with Type 2 diabetes. When this happens, harmful substances known as ketones build up in the body as a result of fat breakdown. This can be life-threatening if you don't seek medical attention straight away.

Symptoms of diabetic ketoacidosis include:

needing to pee more than usual

being sick

pain in the stomach

feeling very thirsty

confusion

breath that smells fruity (people say it smells like pear drops sweets)

feeling very tired

fainting

deep or fast breathing

You can buy home testing kits for diabetic ketoacidosis, which will test your blood or urine for ketones. It's important to call 999 or go to A&E if you are diabetic and worried about the above symptoms.

Diabetes and diet

Healthy eating is a central part of managing diabetes. In some cases, changing your diet may be enough to control the disease.

Type 1 diabetes

Your blood sugar level rises or falls based on the types of foods you eat. Starchy or sugary foods make blood sugar levels rise rapidly. Protein and fat cause more gradual increases.

Your medical team may recommend that you limit the amount of carbohydrates you eat each day. You'll also need to balance your carb intake with your insulin doses.

Work with a dietitian who can help you design a diabetes meal plan. Getting the right balance of protein, fat, and carbs can help you control your blood sugar.

Type 2 diabetes

Eating the right types of foods can both control your blood sugar and help you lose any excess weight.

Carb counting is an important part of eating for type 2 diabetes. A dietitian can help you figure out how many grams of carbohydrates to eat at each meal.

In order to keep your blood sugar levels steady, try to eat small meals throughout the day. Emphasize healthy foods such as:

fruits

vegetables

whole grains

lean protein such as poultry and fish

healthy fats such as olive oil and nuts

Certain other foods can undermine efforts to keep your blood sugar in control. Discover the foods you should avoid if you have diabetes.

Gestational diabetes

Eating a well-balanced diet is important for both you and your baby during these nine months. Making the right food choices can also help you avoid diabetes medications.

Watch your portion sizes, and limit sugary or salty foods. Although you need some sugar to feed your growing baby, you should avoid eating too much.

Consider making an eating plan with the help of a dietitian or nutritionist. They'll ensure that your diet has the right mix of macronutrients. Go here for other do's and don'ts for healthy eating with gestational diabetes.

CHAPTER 2

<u>DIABETES RECIPES</u>

Spiced Sweet Roasted Red Pepper Hummus

<u>Ingredients</u>

1 (15 ounce) can garbanzo beans, drained

1 (4 ounce) jar roasted red peppers

3 tablespoons lemon juice

1 ½ tablespoons tahini

1 clove garlic, minced

½ teaspoon ground cumin

½ teaspoon cayenne pepper

¼ teaspoon salt

1 tablespoon chopped fresh parsley

<u>Directions</u>

Step 1

In an electric blender or food processor, puree the chickpeas, red peppers, lemon juice, tahini, garlic, cumin, cayenne, and salt. Process, using long pulses, until the mixture is fairly smooth, and slightly fluffy. Make sure to scrape the mixture off the sides of the food processor or blender in between pulses. Transfer to a serving bowl and refrigerate for at least 1 hour. (The hummus can be made up to 3 days ahead and refrigerated. Return to room temperature before serving.)

Step 2

Sprinkle the hummus with the chopped parsley before serving.

The Best Dry-Roasted Chickpea Recipe
Ingredient

1 (15 ounce) can garbanzo beans, drained and rinsed

2 teaspoons olive oil

¼ teaspoon salt, or to taste

1 pinch ground black pepper to taste

Directions

Step 1

Preheat oven to 425 degrees F (220 degrees C).

Step 2

Spread garbanzo beans in a baking dish and pat dry with a paper towel.

Step 3

Bake in the preheated oven, stirring halfway through, about 22 minutes. Toss with olive oil, salt, and pepper in a large bowl. Return to the baking dish.

Step 4

Continue baking chickpeas, stirring halfway through, until golden and dry on the outside, about 22 minutes more.

Microwave Corn on the Cob
Ingredients

1 ear corn, husked and cleaned

Directions

Step 1

Wet a paper towel, and wring out. Wrap the ear of corn in the moist towel, and place on a dinner plate. Cook in the microwave for 5 minutes. Carefully remove paper towel, and enjoy!

Easy Apple Coleslaw

Ingredients

3 cups chopped cabbage

1 unpeeled red apple, cored and chopped

1 unpeeled Granny Smith apple, cored and chopped

1 carrot, grated

½ cup finely chopped red bell pepper

2 green onions, finely chopped

⅓ cup mayonnaise

⅓ cup brown sugar

1 tablespoon lemon juice, or to taste

Directions

Step 1

In a large bowl, combine cabbage, red apple, green apple, carrot, red bell pepper, and green onions. In a small bowl, mix together mayonnaise, brown sugar, and lemon juice. Pour dressing over salad.

Red Lentil Curry

Ingredients

2 cups red lentils

1 large onion, diced

1 tablespoon vegetable oil

2 tablespoons curry paste

1 tablespoon curry powder

1 teaspoon ground turmeric

1 teaspoon ground cumin

1 teaspoon chili powder

1 teaspoon salt

1 teaspoon white sugar

1 teaspoon minced garlic

1 teaspoon minced fresh ginger

1 (14.25 ounce) can tomato puree

Directions

Step 1

Wash the lentils in cold water until the water runs clear. Put lentils in a pot with enough water to cover; bring to a boil, place a cover on the pot, reduce heat to medium-low, and simmer, adding water during cooking as needed to keep covered, until tender, 15 to 20 minutes. Drain.

Step 2

Heat vegetable oil in a large skillet over medium heat; cook and stir onions in hot oil until caramelized, about 20 minutes.

Step 3

Mix curry paste, curry powder, turmeric, cumin, chili powder, salt, sugar, garlic, and ginger together in a large bowl; stir into the onions. Increase heat to high and cook, stirring constantly, until fragrant, 1 to 2 minutes.

Step 4

Stir in the tomato puree, remove from heat and stir into the lentils.

Paleo Chicken Stew

Ingredients

2 teaspoons olive oil

1 small red onion, chopped

2 cloves garlic, minced

2 skinless, boneless chicken breast halves, cut into cubes

2 eaches sweet potatoes, peeled and chopped

1 cup fresh spinach, or to taste

1 pinch crushed red pepper, or more to taste

1 pinch paprika, or more to taste

1 pinch sea salt to taste

½ cup chicken broth, or more to taste

Directions

Step 1

Heat olive oil in a saucepan over medium-high heat. Saute onion and garlic in hot oil until softened, about 5 minutes.

Step 2

Stir chicken, sweet potatoes, spinach, crushed red pepper, paprika, and sea salt with the onion and garlic in the saucepan. Pour as much chicken broth into the saucepan to make the mixture as soup-like or stew-like as you'd like it.

Step 3

Bring the broth to a boil, reduce heat to medium-low, and simmer until the chicken is no longer pink in the middle and the sweet potatoes are tender, about 30 minutes.

Mediterranean Kale

<u>Ingredients</u>

12 cups chopped kale

2 tablespoons lemon juice

1 tablespoon olive oil, or as needed

1 tablespoon minced garlic

1 teaspoon soy sauce

salt to taste

ground black pepper to taste

<u>Directions</u>

Step 1

Place a steamer insert into a saucepan, and fill with water to just below the bottom of the steamer. Cover, and bring the water to a boil over high heat. Add the kale, recover, and steam until just tender, 7 to 10 minutes depending on thickness.

Step 2

Whisk together the lemon juice, olive oil, garlic, soy sauce, salt, and black pepper in a large bowl. Toss steamed kale into dressing until well coated.

Grilled Corn Salad

<u>Ingredients</u>

6 ears freshly shucked corn

1 green pepper, diced

2 Roma (plum) tomatoes, diced

¼ cup diced red onion

½ bunch fresh cilantro, chopped, or more to taste

2 teaspoons olive oil, or to taste

1 pinch salt and ground black pepper to taste

<u>Directions</u>

Step 1

Preheat an outdoor grill for medium heat; lightly oil the grate.

Step 2

Cook the corn on the preheated grill, turning occasionally, until the corn is tender and specks of black appear, about 10 minutes; set aside until just cool enough to handle. Slice the kernels off of the cob and place into a bowl.

Step 3

Combine the warm corn kernels with the green pepper, diced tomato, onion, cilantro, and olive oil. Season with salt and pepper; toss until evenly mixed. Set aside for at least 30 minutes to allow flavors to blend before serving.

Autumn Apple Salad II

Ingredients

4 eaches tart green apples, cored and chopped

¼ cup blanched slivered almonds, toasted

¼ cup dried cranberries

¼ cup chopped dried cherries

1 (8 ounce) container vanilla yogurt

Directions

Step 1

In a medium bowl, stir together the apples, almonds, cranberries, cherries and yogurt until evenly coated.

Red, White, and Blueberry Fruit Salad

Ingredients

1 pint strawberries, hulled and quartered

1 pint blueberries

½ cup white sugar

2 tablespoons lemon juice

4 eaches bananas

Directions

Step 1

Mix the strawberries and blueberries together in a bowl, sprinkle with sugar and lemon juice, and toss lightly. Refrigerate until cold, at least 30 minutes. About 30 minutes before serving, cut the bananas into 3/4-inch thick slices, and toss with the berries.

Puerto Rican Tostones (Fried Plantains)

Ingredients

5 tablespoons oil for frying

1 green plantain

3 cups cold water

salt to taste

Directions

Step 1

Peel the plantain and cut it into 1-inch chunks.

Step 2

Heat the oil in a large skillet. Place the plantains in the oil and fry on both sides, approximately 3 1/2 minutes per side.

Step 3

Remove the plantains from the pan and flatten the plantains by placing a plate over the fried plantains and pressing down.

Step 4

Dip the plantains in water, then return them to the hot oil and fry 1 minute on each side. Salt to taste and serve immediately.

Tuscan Style Bean Soup

Ingredients

1 tablespoon olive oil

1 onion, chopped

2 cloves garlic, minced

1 red bell pepper, chopped

3 cups low fat, low sodium chicken broth

1 cup canned whole tomatoes, chopped

1 ½ cups kidney beans, cooked

2 teaspoons chopped fresh thyme

½ cup chopped spinach

1 cup seashell pasta

ground black pepper to taste

Directions

Step 1

In a large pot over medium high heat, combine the oil, onion and garlic and saute for 5 minutes. Add the red bell pepper and saute for 3 more minutes. Add the broth, tomatoes and beans. Bring to a boil, reduce heat to low and simmer for 20 minutes. Add the thyme, spinach and pasta. Simmer for 5 more minutes and pepper to taste.

Easy Roasted Peppers

Ingredients

6 red bell peppers

Directions

Step 1

Preheat the oven to 500 degrees F (260 degrees C).

Step 2

Cut the peppers into quarters. Remove the seeds and the membranes. Roast the peppers until the skin blisters and turns black. Remove from oven and cover with plastic, or a tea towel, or place in a paper bag until cool. The skins should peel away off of the peppers easily when cooled.

Pineapple Salsa

Ingredients

1 cup finely chopped fresh pineapple

½ cup diced red bell pepper

½ cup diced green bell pepper

1 cup frozen corn kernels, thawed

1 (15 ounce) can black beans, drained and rinsed

¼ cup chopped onions

2 green chile peppers, chopped

¼ cup orange juice

¼ cup chopped fresh cilantro

½ teaspoon ground cumin

1 pinch salt and pepper to taste

Directions

Step 1

In a large bowl, toss together pineapple, red bell pepper, green bell pepper, corn, black beans, onions, green chile peppers, orange juice, and cilantro. Season with cumin, salt, and pepper. Cover, and chill in the refrigerator until serving.

Gluten-Free Cheese and Herb Pizza Crust

Ingredients

¾ cup gluten-free all purpose baking flour

¼ cup garbanzo bean flour

¼ cup cornstarch

¼ cup tapioca starch

¼ cup grated Parmesan cheese

1 ½ teaspoons baking powder

1 teaspoon xanthan gum

1 teaspoon Italian seasoning

1 teaspoon dried oregano

½ teaspoon salt

1 teaspoon white sugar

1 cup lukewarm water

1 (.25 ounce) package active dry yeast

1 egg

1 ½ teaspoons olive oil

½ teaspoon apple cider vinegar

1 teaspoon white sugar

½ teaspoon minced garlic

Directions

Step 1

Preheat oven to 425 degrees F (220 degrees C). Grease a 15-inch pizza pan with cooking spray.

Step 2

Stir all-purpose baking flour, garbanzo bean flour, cornstarch, tapioca starch, Parmesan cheese, baking powder, xanthan gum, Italian seasoning, oregano, and salt together in a bowl; set aside.

Step 3

Dissolve 1 teaspoon of white sugar in lukewarm water in a small bowl. Sprinkle yeast over top, and set aside until foamy, 3 to 5 minutes.

Step 4

Beat egg in a separate bowl with olive oil, vinegar, 1 teaspoon sugar, and garlic until smooth. Whisk yeast mixture into egg mixture and stir in flour mixture until no dry lumps remain. Press dough into prepared pan, leaving outer edge slightly thicker than the center.

Step 5

Cook in preheated oven until dough has risen and slightly firmed, 10 to 12 minutes.

Step 6

Once topped with your favorite toppings, continue baking at 425 degrees F (220 degrees C) until the crust is golden brown, 20 to 30 minutes. Remove pizza from pan and cook directly on the oven rack for 5 minutes to crisp crust, if desired.

Fruit Skewers with Apple Cinnamon Dipping Sauce

Ingredients

½ cup vanilla Greek-style yogurt

2 tablespoons applesauce (such as Mott's® Natural Applesauce)

⅛ teaspoon almond extract

⅛ teaspoon ground cinnamon

1 cup seedless grapes

1 cup fresh strawberries

1 cup apple chunks

1 cup pineapple chunks

8 (6 inch) wooden skewers

Directions

Step 1

Stir yogurt, applesauce, almond extract, and cinnamon together in a bowl until dipping sauce is well-combined.

Step 2

Thread grapes, strawberries, apple chunks, and pineapple chunks alternatively onto skewers. Arrange finished skewers on a plate and serve with dipping sauce.

Penne Pasta with Simple Beef Neck Sauce

Ingredients

3 pounds beef neck bones

1 onion, cut into chunks

3 cups tomato sauce, or more to taste

1 cup water, or more as needed

1 tablespoon chopped fresh parsley, or to taste

1 tablespoon chopped fresh oregano, or to taste

1 pinch red pepper flakes, or to taste

salt and freshly ground black pepper to taste

1 pound penne pasta, or to taste

¼ cup grated Parmesan cheese, or to taste

Directions

Step 1

Preheat oven to 400 degrees F (200 degrees C). Spread neck bones and onions out in the bottom of a roasting pan.

Step 2

Roast in the preheated oven until bones are browned and caramelized, 45 minutes.

Step 3

Combine beef and onions, tomato sauce, and water in a large pot; bring to a simmer, reduce heat to low, and simmer, skimming fat and adding water as needed, until meat is falling off the bones, about 6 hours.

Step 4

Stir parsley, oregano, red pepper flakes, salt, and ground black pepper into tomato sauce mixture; simmer until flavors combine, 10 to 15 minutes.

Step 5

Bring a large pot of lightly salted water to a boil; add penne and cook, stirring occasionally, until tender yet firm to the bite, about 11 minutes. Drain.

Step 6

Stir penne and 1/2 of the sauce together in a bowl with some of the Parmesan cheese. Spoon into bowls and top with remaining sauce and Parmesan cheese.

Eskimo Cubes for Summer

Ingredients

2 ½ cups cubed seeded watermelon

2 ½ cups cubed cantaloupe

2 ½ cups cubed honeydew

1 cup frozen raspberries, thawed

1 cup frozen strawberries, thawed

¼ cup white sugar

1 tablespoon lemon juice

Directions

Step 1

Blend the watermelon, cantaloupe, honeydew, raspberries, strawberries, sugar, and lemon juice in a blender until smooth.

Step 2

Pour the blended fruit juice into molds and cover with aluminum foil; poke a stick into the center. Store in freezer until frozen through, about 4 hours.

Vegetarian 15-Bean Soup

Ingredients

1 (20 ounce) package 15-bean soup mix (seasoning packet not used)

2 tablespoons olive oil, or more as needed

1 large onion, diced

12 carrots, peeled and chopped, or more to taste

15 crimini mushrooms, sliced, or more to taste

7 stalks celery, chopped, or more to taste

6 leaves dinosaur kale, chopped

4 leaves red Swiss chard, chopped

3 large cloves garlic, minced

12 cups vegetable broth

2 bay leaves

1 teaspoon dried rosemary

1 teaspoon dried basil

1 pinch salt and ground black pepper to taste

<u>Directions</u>

Step 1

Place beans in a large container and cover with several inches of cool water; let stand 8 hours to overnight. Drain and rinse.

Step 2

Heat olive oil in a stockpot over medium heat; cook and stir onion until golden brown, 15 to 20 minutes. Add carrots, mushrooms, celery, kale, chard, and garlic; cook

and stir until carrots and mushrooms are slightly tender,
5 to 10 minutes.

Step 3

Pour broth over vegetable mixture and bring to a boil;
reduce heat and add bay leaves, rosemary, basil, salt, and
pepper. Add beans and simmer soup until beans are
softened, 1 1/2 to 2 hours.

Roasted and Pickled Beets

Ingredients

12 small beets

3 tablespoons balsamic vinegar

2 tablespoons honey

1 tablespoon red wine vinegar

1 pinch salt and ground black pepper to taste

½ cup thinly sliced onion

Directions

Step 1

Preheat oven to 400 degrees F (200 degrees C). Place
beets in a shallow pan.

Step 2

Roast beets in the preheated oven until tender, about 1 hour. Remove pan from oven and cool beets until easily handled, at least 15 minutes.

Step 3

Peel beets and cut into 1/4-inch-thick slices.

Step 4

Beat balsamic vinegar, honey, and red wine vinegar together with a whisk in a bowl until dressing is smooth.

Step 5

Mix beets and onion in a bowl. Drizzle dressing over beet mixture and toss to coat; refrigerate until chilled, about 1 hour.

Panzanella

Ingredients

5 cups chopped tomato

1 cup chopped cucumber

½ cup sliced green onions

½ cup chopped sweet yellow pepper

½ cup chopped fresh parsley

¼ cup chopped fresh basil leaves

¼ cup fresh lemon juice

1 ½ tablespoons olive oil

¼ teaspoon ground black pepper

1 garlic clove, minced

4 cups cubed French bread

Directions

Step 1

In a large bowl, combine tomatoes, cucumber, green onion, yellow pepper, parsley, and basil.

Step 2

In a small bowl, whisk together lemon juice, olive oil, salt, ground black pepper, and garlic. Pour lemon juice mixture over the tomato mixture, and toss to coat. Refrigerate for 30 minutes.

Step 3

Meanwhile, preheat oven to 350 degrees F (175 degrees C). Place bread cubes in a single layer on a baking sheet. Bake for 12 minutes, or until toasted and dry.

Step 4

Toss bread cubes with tomato mixture, and serve.

Lentils in Sloppy Joe Sauce

Ingredients

1 tablespoon oil, or as needed

½ onion, minced

½ green bell pepper, minced

2 tablespoons minced garlic

1 cup water

¾ cup ketchup

3 tablespoons spicy brown mustard

2 tablespoons soy sauce

2 tablespoons barbeque sauce

1 tablespoon maple syrup

1 tablespoon sriracha hot sauce

1 teaspoon thyme

1 teaspoon cayenne pepper, or to taste

2 cups cooked lentils, or more to taste

Directions

Step 1

Heal oil in a deep skillet over medium heat; cook and stir onion, green bell pepper, and garlic until until tender, about 10 minutes. Add water, ketchup, brown mustard, soy sauce, barbeque sauce, maple syrup, sriracha hot sauce, thyme, and cayenne pepper to onion mixture; bring to a boil.

Step 2

Reduce heat to medium and simmer until sauce is thickened, about 5 minutes. Stir lentils into sauce and simmer until lentils are warmed, about 5 minutes.

Super Spinach Salad

**Ingredients**

2 cups packed fresh spinach

½ cup cooked quinoa

¼ cup shredded carrots

¼ cup dried cranberries

¼ cup canned chickpeas (garbanzo beans)

¼ cup edamame (green soybeans)

2 tablespoons pumpkin seeds

¼ cup ginger-miso dressing, or to taste

<u>Directions</u>

 Step 1

Combine spinach, quinoa, carrots, cranberries, chickpeas, edamame, and pumpkin seeds in a bowl; add dressing and toss to coat.

Lemon Pound Cake with Lemon Glaze

<u>Ingredients</u>

1 cup unsalted butter

½ cup Pyure Organic All Purpose Stevia Blend

4 eggs

1 teaspoon vanilla extract

1 tablespoon finely grated lemon zest

1 ¾ cups all-purpose flour

1 teaspoon baking powder

½ teaspoon baking soda

½ teaspoon salt

3 tablespoons milk

Lemon Glaze:

⅓ cup lemon juice

½ cup Pyure Organic All Purpose Stevia Blend

½ teaspoon Pyure Organic Liquid Stevia Extract - Simply
Sweet

Directions

Step 1

Preheat oven to 325 degrees F. Line an 8 x 4-inch loaf pan
with parchment paper and set aside.

Step 2

Beat together butter and Pyure Organic All Purpose
Stevia Blend until fluffy. Add eggs, one at a time, blending
after each addition. Beat in vanilla and lemon zest.

Step 3

Whisk together flour, baking powder, baking soda and
salt. Stir flour mixture into butter mixture, alternating
with milk.

Step 4

Scrape batter into prepared pan. Bake for 50 to 55
minutes or until tester inserted into center comes out
clean. Let stand 5 minutes. Remove cake from pan and
let cool on rack.

Step 5

Lemon Glaze: Add water to lemon juice to bring up to 1/2 cup. Combine in saucepan with Pyure Organic All Purpose Stevia Blend and Pyure Organic Liquid Stevia. Bring to a boil on medium and cook for 8 to 10 minutes or until slightly thickened and reduced by two-thirds.

Step 6

Brush glaze over cooled cake.

Honeysuckle Pineapple

Ingredients

4 slices fresh pineapple

1 ½ tablespoons honey

2 tablespoons cherry brandy

1 teaspoon lemon juice

Directions

Step 1

To Marinate: Combine honey, brandy and lemon juice in a nonporous glass dish or bowl. Mix together and add pineapple; coat well with marinade mixture. Cover dish and marinate in refrigerator for 1 hour.

Step 2

Preheat grill to medium heat and lightly oil grate.

Step 3

Remove pineapple from dish or bowl, discarding any
leftover marinade. Place pineapple wedges directly on
rack or in a basket and grill for about 10 minutes, turning,
until pineapple is hot and caramelized.

Lactose Free Corn Chowder
<u>Ingredients</u>

5 medium (2-1/4" to 3" dia, raw)s potatoes, peeled and
cubed

1 cup chopped celery

½ cup sliced leeks

½ cup chopped green onions

2 cups fresh corn kernels

1 tablespoon dried parsley

1 cup non-dairy creamer

salt and pepper to taste

Directions

Step 1

In a 3 quart pot over high heat, combine the potatoes with enough water to cover. Boil for one hour, adding water to cover potatoes as necessary. Add the celery, leeks and scallions and boil for another hour.

Step 2

Reduce heat to low, add the corn and parsley and heat through. Add the non-dairy creamer just before serving. Enjoy!

Freezer Slaw

Ingredients

1 large head cabbage, shredded

1 green bell pepper, finely chopped

1 small small onion, finely chopped

2 carrots, shredded

2 cups boiling water

2 teaspoons salt

1 ½ cups white sugar

1 cup water

¾ cup cider vinegar

2 teaspoons celery seed

Directions

Step 1

Combine cabbage, green bell pepper, onion, and carrots in a large bowl. Mix boiling water and salt together in a bowl and pour over cabbage mixture. Set aside for salt to draw out extra water from vegetables, about 1 hour. Drain well.

Step 2

Mix sugar, 1 cup water, cider vinegar, and celery seed in a saucepan; bring to a boil. Cook and stir until sugar is dissolved, about 1 minute. Remove saucepan from heat and cool completely.

Step 3

Pour cooled sugar-vinegar mixture over drained cabbage mixture in a large bowl and toss until slaw is well mixed. Spoon slaw into resealable plastic bags and freeze.

Grandma's Carrot Salad

Ingredients

1 pound shredded carrots

1 ¼ cups raisins

2 tablespoons mayonnaise, or to taste

1 teaspoon lemon juice

¼ teaspoon salt

<u>**Directions**</u>

Step 1

Mix carrots and raisins together in a large bowl. Whisk mayonnaise, lemon juice, and salt together in a small bowl until smooth. Pour lemon juice mixture over carrot mixture and stir until carrots are completely coated. Refrigerate until chilled, at least 30 minutes.

Vegan French Toast
<u>**Ingredients**</u>

1 cup soy milk

2 tablespoons all-purpose flour

1 tablespoon nutritional yeast

1 teaspoon raw sugar

1 teaspoon vanilla extract

⅓ teaspoon ground cinnamon

4 slices bread

Directions

Step 1

Whisk soy milk, flour, nutritional yeast, sugar, vanilla extract, and cinnamon together in a bowl; transfer to a rimmed plate or shallow dish. Dip both sides of each bread slice in soy milk mixture.

Step 2

Heat a lightly oiled skillet over medium-low heat. Cook each slice of bread until golden brown, 3 to 4 minutes per side.

Baked Potato

Ingredients

1 baking potato

Directions

Step 1

Preheat oven to 350 degrees F (175 degrees C).

Step 2

Scrub the potato and prick it with a fork to prevent steam from building up and causing the potato to explode in your oven.

 Step 3

Bake for 1 1/2 hours.

Date Haroset

Ingredients

½ pound chopped dates

1 cup golden raisins

½ cup red wine

½ cup coarsely chopped walnuts

1 teaspoon ground cinnamon

½ cup confectioners' sugar

Directions

 Step 1

Place the chopped dates and golden raisins in a small saucepan with the wine. Cook over low heat, stirring occasionally, until the fruit thickens to a soft paste. Cool.

Step 2

Stir nuts and cinnamon into the cooled fruit mixture.

Step 3

Form paste into small, bite-size balls. Roll in confectioners' sugar.

Banana Oat and Bran Cookies
<u>Ingredients</u>

2 ripe bananas, mashed

½ cup whole wheat flour

¼ cup wheat bran

¼ cup rolled oats

½ cup packed brown sugar

½ cup low-fat plain yogurt

⅛ cup real maple syrup

2 egg whites

1 teaspoon ground cinnamon

½ teaspoon salt

½ teaspoon baking powder

½ cup raisins

Directions

Step 1

Preheat oven to 350 degrees F (175 degrees C).

Step 2

Beat mashed bananas, egg whites, brown sugar, maple syrup, yogurt, and cinnamon.

Step 3

Combine the remaining dry ingredients: flour, oats, wheat bran, salt and baking powder in a separate bowl. Use an electric mixer to combine dry ingredients with wet mixture.

Step 4

Add in raisins, chopped prunes, and/ or nuts.

Step 5

Roll cookies into balls, place on a cookie sheet coated with cooking spray. Bake for 8-12 minutes until cookies are firm and dry.

No Bake Bumpy Peanut Butter Nuggets

Ingredients

½ cup natural peanut butter

¼ cup nonfat dry milk powder

¼ cup unsweetened flaked coconut

⅓ cup rolled oats

½ teaspoon ground cinnamon

¼ cup wheat germ

¼ cup unsweetened apple juice concentrate, thawed

Directions

Step 1

Combine peanut butter, milk powder, and coconut in a large mixing bowl. Stir in oats, ground cinnamon, wheat germ, and apple juice concentrate until thoroughly combined.

Step 2

Shape the mixture into 1 inch balls. Chill thoroughly before serving; store remaining nuggets in the refrigerator.

Chicken Vegetable Stew

Ingredients

4 skinless, boneless chicken breast halves, cut into bite size pieces

1 onion, chopped

½ pound baby carrots

4 medium (2-1/4" to 3" dia, raw)s potatoes

½ teaspoon salt

¼ teaspoon ground turmeric

3 tablespoons tomato paste

½ cup water

¼ teaspoon garlic powder

½ teaspoon ground black pepper

Directions

Step 1

In a large pot, put the chopped onion, chicken breast meat, carrots and potatoes. Add the salt and turmeric. Dissolve the tomato paste in water and add. If desired, add garlic powder and ground black pepper to season.

Step 2

Cook for 1 to 1 1/2 hours on medium low heat. Serve.

Popcorn Macaroons
Ingredients

2 cups popped popcorn

3 egg whites

½ teaspoon baking powder

¼ teaspoon salt

¼ teaspoon cream of tartar

2 tablespoons granulated artificial sweetener

Directions

Step 1

Preheat oven to 350 degrees F (175 degrees C). Lightly grease cookie sheets. Place popped popcorn into a food processor or blender; grind into small kernels.

Step 2

In a large bowl, whip egg whites until frothy. Add baking powder, salt and cream of tartar; continue whipping to stiff peaks. Gradually mix in the sugar substitute. Fold in the popcorn pieces. Drop by teaspoonfuls onto the prepared cookie sheets.

Step 3

Bake for 12 to 15 minutes in the preheated oven, or until lightly browned. Allow cookies to cool on cookie sheets before removing.

CONCLUSION

Some types of diabetes — like type 1 — are caused by factors that are out of your control. Others — like type 2 — can be prevented with better food choices, increased activity, and weight loss.

Discuss potential diabetes risks with your doctor. If you're at risk, have your blood sugar tested and follow your doctor's advice for managing your blood sugar.